FEELING
GOOD YOU

The Art of Catching
The Exercise High

Jim Ringers

For permissions contact: info@jimringers.com

Publishing Services provided by Paper Raven Books LLC

Printed in the United States of America

First Printing, 2022

Paperback ISBN: 979-8-4610713-2-5

Disclaimer

The author and publisher of this eBook and the accompanying materials have used their best efforts in preparing this eBook. The author and publisher make no representation or warranties with respect to the accuracy, applicability, fitness, or completeness of this eBook's contents. The information contained in this eBook is strictly for educational purposes. Therefore, if you wish to apply the ideas contained in this eBook, you are taking full responsibility for your actions.

Table of Contents

Introduction

Feelinggoodyou aka Superfragicajilistic, Great, Pure, Righteous, High, Soaring Spirits is a spirit-based health and fitness program designed for people at all levels who would like to know how to get healthy without having to go to a gym or spend a whole lot of money on a diet program. We will do 80% of our exercise program with just a simple mat. So, you don't have to leave the comfort of your own home. We will start with the simplest of remedies and exercises for Joe Six-Pack, and Jo Chardonnay and slowly make our way up the mountain for those who are interested in elite fitness. It won't be long for you to be feeling good and looking good!

Any recommendations I may make about weight training, nutrition, supplements or lifestyle, should be discussed between you and your doctor or other relevant licensed professional because exercising involves risks. The information you receive on this website or in person or any form does not take the place of medical advice. Before starting any exercise program, please check with your doctor or other relevant licensed professional, and clear any exercises and/or diet changes with them before starting any such regimen. I am not a doctor, nutritionist or registered dietician. I do not claim to help cure any condition or disease.

Free Gift

Get a FREE step by step beginner friendly guide to Losing Weight, Feeling Good and Looking Great.

Don't miss out. Start Feeling Good now!

Get the Free Guide right here!

https://access.feelinggoodyou.com/free

Where FeelingGoodYou Began

I'd like to start with a story about this program's origin's; where it all began. When I was 21 years old, I dove into shallow water and fractured my 5th and 6th vertebrae. As a result, I was paralyzed from the waist down and unable to walk. After a few weeks, I took my first steps and was on the road to a recovery that was pretty much hopeless. It is incredible what the spine governs in the body. If you didn't know, it's just about everything, including strength, flexibility, balance, and coordination among others. Looking back, the most affected thing was my spirit. It was crushed, and I didn't believe I would ever regain any spirit, energy, and belief in my abilities.

Strangely enough, I don't think I can recognize the person I was before the accident. It's almost as if I was a different person in a different life. As I emerged into this new life, I headed down a very dark path, where feeling good meant taking a pill or a drink. I'm really not sure what turned me around; maybe, it was surfing? I thought a wave could wash away any hangover.

When I went for my first surf/boogie board adventure in California near Huntington Beach, it was no joke. The waves were pretty big, and I had no idea what I was doing. I did have a couple friends (I referred to them as "brohams") that sort of showed me how to paddle out, and they showed me the path to take along the rocks. I made my way out to the waves, after some tricky navigating. But, since I didn't know anything about catching waves; I was pummeled by the big waves, and walked away sort of beaten.

Years later, I arrived in Daytona Beach, Florida. Here the waves were not so big, and I was able to not only boogie board, but I was able to start learning to surf too!! I coined my favorite wave as "two feet and glassy" which I was more apt to find early in the morning. This smaller wave was ideal for learning!

Why did I feel so good during and after surfing? I think the first most obvious answer is by going swimming and immersing yourself in water, you're just going to feel good. Taking a shower makes you feel good. And that's why I made showering an important step in my Free Guide "Catching the Exercise High."

What else is there about surfing that showed me how to feel good? And how can I take that and apply it to a ten minute or thirty minute workout at home? That was the question? One of the things I learned from surfing was that it's important to be a good swimmer. As I began to take up lap swimming I noticed I would get the same euphoric feeling after the swim that I got after surfing. The doctors/scholars can look at brain waves on an EEG(electroencephalogram), and see what they look like after swimming. So with surfing and swimming I like to say you're not only catching waves; you're catching "brain waves". The five brain waves the scholars talk about are Gamma, Beta, Alpha, Theta and Delta. Delta waves are your sleeping, deep dreaming, waves. Theta waves are the waves before your deep sleep. Alpha waves are the waves that we are trying to produce through moderate exercise. I refer to them as the feel good waves, and others refer to them as the waves that are best for learning, problem solving, and sports performance, sort of a relaxed, satisfied state, or the flow state. Beta waves are the waves we use for our day to day activities and our awake state, or open eyed state in order to get things done. But the Beta wave state loses when it comes to optimum performance. So for our day to day activities in order to perform our best, and feel our best, we can consciously change our brain waves from Beta to Alpha waves. Gamma waves are your fastest moving waves and used for heavy concentration. I'm not a brain wave specialist, but I believe swimming produces brain waves that make you feel good, and to some extent perform better.

When jumping on a surfboard one of the things that hits you immediately is the sounds of nature. It has been documented that listening to nature sounds has a powerful effect on mood. You start with the sound of the ocean waves. This rolling sound may wash away the pain and troubles from your brain. While surfing there are other sounds that you are keenly aware of: the sound of birds, the sound of the wind, the sounds of fish jumping out of the water. It reminds me of Native American Indian Chief Dan George who wrote, *My Spirit Soars*. When he walked in the deep woods, he heard the sounds of nature and spoke to the animals and wrote of his soaring spirit!. I believe his mood was affected by the natural sounds around him. Similarly with surfing you are immersed in nature, and this helps your spirit soar.

What else about surfing showed me how to feel good? I feel that the exercise you get from surfing is second to none. Simply walking in the surf can be an amazing workout requiring muscles and balance you never used before. If you miss any muscles you will need to use those while you are out surfing in the deeper water. Surfing helps your balance, and balance is important in many sports. Greg Norman "The Shark" an old school golfer, who grew up in Australia, credited surfing for his superior balance and successful golf career. Having good balance is a gift, and surfing builds good balance naturally. Using all these different muscles is one of the reasons why I like to encourage others to exercise using many different disciplines. I think it stimulates your coordination. I also believe that variety with your exercise helps you catch the "exercise high" to a greater degree.

Now that I'm away from the beach, and live in a city, I still make it a point to swim at least once a week. I think there is a lot of value in swimming. To put it more simply, swimming makes you feel good. And when I'm at the pool I ask people after they swim. How do you feel, or how was your swim? And seemingly all the people enthusiastically respond that they feel great; and that they love the way they feel after a swim.

Jack Lalanne was a big fan of swimming. Jack Lalanne towed 70 boats handcuffed and shackled on his 70 birthday by using the dolphin kick which is the butterfly kick.

Performing the butterfly is a great way to kick in the feel good endorphins. And there is no question that I feel extra good after just one lap of the butterfly. I believe I can fly…

Surfing not only taught me how to feel good, it taught me to fly. I felt the exercise high in full force. As time marched by, I began swimming for exercise and gave martial arts a try. The simplest way to describe what was wrong with me was that I was missing a few batteries in my body, mind, and spirit. I needed to recharge my body, and I felt that a workout would give me the electrical shock I needed. It was almost like how someone having a heart attack gets shocked back into life. Through it all, I learned how to lose weight, gain balance, strength, and coordination, and live a more fulfilling life. I attained a CSCS certificate from the NSCA for Personal Training and eventually earned my black belt in BJJ. The best examples I can think of for a healthy lifestyle are Jack LaLanne and Paul & Patricia Bragg. They possessed uncontained joy, enthusiasm and a zest for life. This is what we want to ignite and give life to. And hopefully, make it simple and easy.

Many years ago, I read a poem titled *The Beauty of the Trees*, by Dan George, a Native American chief, and a well-known actor known for his appearance with Clint Eastwood in the film Outlaw Josey Wales. After reading this poem, I began thinking. His poem was basically about his walks in the woods. Whenever, he would listen to the wind, or watch an eagle fly, his spirit or heart would soar. To my sorrow, my thought was that my spirit doesn't soar, certainly not with a walk in the woods. My spirit may soar while I am making money? I did think about times when my spirit may have soared, but we called it endorphins or adrenaline rush? Catching a wave on a surfboard seemed like a good time at first. Running my hand across the wall of a wave years later was a little different; I felt the endorphins or the exercise high; I might say, "my spirit soared!" Another random encounter I had with the feel-good spirit was hiking up a rock in Phoenix, AZ. As I was walking up the rock, I noticed my heart was pounding through my chest. I'm not a big hiker, but I assumed that this rock's elevation was enough to get my heart pumping. When I reached the summit, it was getting dark, and the lights of the city made for an epic view. Here, the feel-good spirit left its mark in my memory. I also remember diving into home plate as a kid for an in-the-park home run. That also sparked the exercise high and had me feeling good. I started developing this program after spending a few years in a martial arts gym. At which point, I was over

50 years old and had sustained a shoulder injury. Was I also chronically overweight even after training every other day for two-hour sessions? I referred to my look as "Shlobby," (a made-up word that combined "fat" and "slobby."). With all the exercise I did, I was constantly hungry, and I was always eating. Now that I was on the sidelines, my focus was to get in shape, lose some weight, become stronger, improve my flexibility, and increase my endurance. After an undetermined amount of time, my real focus began to be "catching the spirit" or getting the exercise high, which seemed to be allusive at times. There were many times I walked out of the martial arts gym with a soaring spirit, wondering if I could replicate that with basic functional fitness?

What were the common factors in the things that I did that gave me the exercise high, before? Maybe it was a rapid heart rate, heavy breathing, maybe a dash of victory?

What I remember as a martial arts practitioner immediately after a sparring session is clearly thinking in astonishment that every single pore was wide open. And that's when I recognized the spirit or, "the fix". I also would typically have a high spirit as I jumped in the car and drove home, especially if I had a decent day in the gym. If things didn't go so well, maybe I'd feel better next time. Getting submitted by a lower belt can definitely take the wind out of your sails. That's a downer.

Now, let's share a couple of thoughts on exercise. Who wants to exercise? Most people don't like to exercise. Who wants to exercise when they can hang out on the couch and watch TV eating a bag of Doritos? That seems a lot more fun. And truth be told, exercising doesn't guarantee that you will look or feel better. There are many ways of exercising that can cause excruciating pain. You may get stronger and build your endurance if you keep at it, but if you don't control your diet, there is no guarantee that you will lose any weight, look any better or, for that matter, get healthy. You may look Shlobby? And finally, who has the time for exercise? Traveling to a gym, exercising, and coming back could easily take three hours? So, where do we begin?

The Path of Least Resistance

What we need in this situation is a magic bullet. The magic bullet—drum roll please—hit the tambourine…**simply fasting**. This is our first step up the mountain. It's also our foundation. You might wonder if there is any scientific proof behind the effectiveness of fasting. The short answer is, "Yes there is!"

Fasting is a marvel for health and fitness. There are many different ways to fast. And I encourage you to research fasting. It's been around for a long time and mentioned in every Holy Book that I can think of? Hippocrates, the father of medicine, recommended fasting. The fast I recommend is the 24-hr. fast once or twice a week. It is a fast from food, not water. Drink filtered water or the best mountain water you can find. Some people prefer distilled water when they fast. There are a few things to consider when choosing the best water for your health, among the many factors is the way the water is stored.

Fasting will be your secret to losing fat. At times you may feel hungry or uncomfortable, but your first bite of food after 24-hrs. will taste greaaaat, and will be well worth the wait. You will appreciate your food more and have a sense of thanksgiving after a day of fasting. Fasting is the path of least resistance. To think you can sit on the couch and lose weight? It can also save you money and time.

You're not buying any weight loss supplements or programs. You're saving money on food! You don't have to do any dishes. There is also a spiritual component to fasting as you will need to have a little endurance and some will. And after about 18 hours your sense of smell will increase and your sense of taste will multiply. And when you sit down to your first meal, your spirit will soar. And finally, fasting is more effective for losing weight than exercise. Why spend hours in the gym if you are not going to control your diet?

Wake up! I have to throw some passion in here because this is the secret to your health!

Start with once a week for a month and after four successful fasts, you will be realizing this really is not that hard. Stick with it for the second month. By the end of the third month, you will see and feel the difference and you will begin to believe in a new you.

You may decide to feed the fire and begin fasting twice a week; by the end of six months, you will need a tailor. If you would like to read about all the medical documentation, I recommend the book *Eat Stop Eat*, by Brad Pilon. This book will go in-depth about the documentation behind the effectiveness of fasting. It will also answer any questions you may have about fasting and give you tips about how to lead a successful fast. *The Miracle of Fasting*, by Paul Bragg N.D., Ph.D. and Patricia Bragg N.D., Ph.D. is also a good read and can help you get started with longer fasts. With fasting alone, you will look great and feel great too! And I believe if you follow this path you will live life more abundantly.

If you are struggling with fasting don't give up. The battle is really all between your ears. Your body and mind will fight against you, and in the beginning, throw its best hunger pangs your way. You need to simply rise up and defeat the hunger pangs and believe that you can skip a meal or two: drink water, green or black tea, or black coffee to fight the hunger pangs or exercise and simply go for a walk. If you can't complete the 24-hr. fast, try again in a couple of days or next week.

Write down the length of your fasting time, and try to beat it the next time. It will not take long to hit the 24-hr. mark. With time the pangs will be much less and you will begin to look forward to your days of fasting. Especially when you see the results!

If you start enjoying fasting and its many benefits, and you start taking on longer fasts, take your time moving up the ladder and gradually extending your fasts. For anything over a five-day fast, seek professional advice and supervision. Some people claim that extended fasts help them reach some sort of an epiphany or that they find freedom and emancipation. It grants freedom from doing dishes for sure. However, keep in mind, the science from Brad Pilon's research supports the 24-hr. fast as the most effective, and the easiest to stick to on a long-term basis.

To be honest, I eventually turned the 24-hour fast into a 23 or 22-hour fast. It just made it a lot easier to keep dinner at the same time. I also typically eat twice a day 12:00 (noon) and 7:30 pm. I think the experts recommend eight hours between meals, but this is what I do. I'm typically just not hungry in the morning. And once or twice a week I fast and eat once a day. If you read up on, "intermittent fasting" you can come up with a myriad of different ways to fast. But this is what works for me.

I'd like to add that with all the diets out there, I have to laugh at how simple and effective this one is. When you start getting used to fasting, it just seems so natural... as if we were designed to go without food for an extended period of time?

Gandhi said this about fasting, "A genuine fast cleanses the body, mind, and soul. It crucifies the flesh and to that extent sets the soul free."

Nutrition in Addition to Fasting

I'm not a nutritionist. However, I can offer some basic advice from my perspective and personal research. The bottom line when it comes to diets is that if you want to trim down, don't overeat. It is important to chew your food. I'm not going to tell you how many bites you need to take when you're eating, however, the more bites or the longer the food is in your mouth the easier it is for your body to digest. I believe in *superfoods*, e.g., garlic, blueberries, watermelon, olive oil.

There are a lot more out there. Fruits and vegetables, herbs, and spices are all important for your energy. If you are not familiar with herbs and spices and their potential to affect your health search, "10 herbs and spices that can help you feel good." That's a good start.

I like Mediterranean diets and things that have been around for a long time. Have a balanced diet. Make sure you are getting your Vitamin C. It's best to get it naturally with oranges, lemons, and tangerines, among other sources but taking the Vitamin C tablet is good in a pinch. And my favorite health cocktail from the great Paul & Patricia Bragg is distilled water, apple cider vinegar, and a little natural honey. Also, try practicing the old saying, "an apple a day keeps the doctor away." To climb higher up the mountain consider the vegan lifestyle, and plant based foods.

To find out more about nutrition check out the suggested books at the end.

I am not endorsing the advice the reader may find in any of these books, but I found the books personally helpful. Any person buying or reading a suggested book should consult with a health professional before beginning any changes in diet and exercise.

Staying on the Path of Least Resistance with Breathing

How do we breathe while exercising? For starters it's important to mention that spirit in Latin means breath. Some say when God formed man he breathed through his nostrils and gave him a spirit.

Let's just start by saying it's important to breathe through your nose. Breathe out through your nose too. John Douillard's book *Body, Mind, & Sport* goes into detail about nose breathing while exercising.

I encourage you to pick up a copy of his book and spend the time mastering this technique. Specifically, the Darth Vader technique. The Darth Vader breath is achieved by making the Ha sound while trying to warm up your hands or fog a mirror, but do it with your mouth closed and breathe through your nose. You will feel the sound in your throat. You can also make this sound on the inhale, but as your exercise intensity increases it becomes difficult to do. As the intensity increases you are encouraged to make the Ha sound only on the exhale. The author was a world-class triathlete and used this technique to improve his performance! Don't expect to start winning races while breathing through your nose right away. Typically, if you need to breathe through your mouth, slow **down your exercise** (type Z personality types will like this part about slowing down the exercise).

If you need to slow down during exercise, stop, take fifteen to thirty deep breaths through your nose. Do a simple stretch while catching your breath, or sit down American Indian style. Rest until your breathing is slow and relaxed. As you are stretching or just sitting to recover, take note of your breaths. If you are keeping the right pace your breath should feel like an automatic pump in perfect synchronicity. If you are struggling to catch your breath you are exercising too vigorously.

Another little tip on helping your breathing: start playing a wind instrument, e.g., a harmonica, etc. I like the harmonica because it's inexpensive and it's easy to carry around, and while playing you are exhaling and inhaling to play music which helps work those breathing muscles. Maybe you want to play the saxophone, the flute, or some bagpipes; even just singing will give you all the benefits you can garner from a wind instrument, and playing or performing music helps you feel good.

You don't need to be a talented musician to blow through your harmonica until you cannot hear any more notes. That will be a complete exhale; now breathe in through your nose. Feel and see your chest rise. Do that a few times and you will be stretching your thoracic cavity and strengthening your lungs. Don't get bogged down because you are not making music; rather think of it simply as an exercise for your lungs and some stomach muscles you've never felt before. In time you will surprise yourself, and maybe reap a little joy and satisfaction playing a simple tune. The point is, your lungs are really the secret to life. Any yogi will tell you so.

Getting Organizizzzzed!!

First Things First

Before starting any exercise program, you should consult with your physician. Let your physician know that you would like to begin doing moderate exercise and would like a check-up. Your doctor will check your weight and your blood pressure among other things. Please ask that they check your cholesterol too. And write down your resting heart rate because you will need that to calculate your target exercise heart rate. They will most likely take a blood sample and run all kinds of tests. At this time, you can also take hip and chest measurements. Put all this information on an index card and store it in a safe place. You will be glad to look at these notes in a few months after you have successfully lost some weight and trimmed down.

Getting Started with a Mat or a Magic Carpet

It's good to think big so let's start with an oversized mat—the thicker, the better. Most yoga mats are pretty thin. My yoga mats are 1/2" thick, and I have another matt underneath that is 1/8" thick. I like to have something underneath my yoga mat like an exercise mat or a carpet. Carve out an area that gives you plenty of room to do a few exercises. You will need to find an area in your apartment or bedroom, yard, or garage with the dimensions of approximately 6' x 9'. If you can afford to get an exercise mat to fill this area, great. If not, a rug or blanket should suffice to get you started. Maybe tape a few yoga mats together or even some cardboard to help cushion the area. When you take a seat on the mat it should feel comfortable.

A friend of mine used the 1' by 1' interlocking squares that are 1" thick, and the mat was approximately 12' x 12'. It was exceptionally nice.

Exercise Equipment

To climb up the mountain of fitness you can get by with just the mat. Keep your mat clean daily with water and vinegar, and when possible exercise with long sleeves and long pants. The less contact your body has with the mat the better. A perfect exercise outfit is a long underwear, top, and bottom.

It would be best to purchase a 10 lb. kettlebell, a pull-up bar, a jump rope, a 16 oz. water bottle, and a baseball bat to get started. Keep it simple!

For starters, you'll need five illustrated books to help you follow along the path. The five books are:

- *The Genius of Flexibility* by Bob Cooley
- *Yoga: The Iyengar Way* by Silva, Mira & Shyam Mehta
- *The New York City Ballet Workout* by Peter Martins
- *The Pilates Powerhouse* by Mari Winsor
- *The Qigong Bible* by Katherine Allen

All these books are illustrated books and all you need to do is turn the page and follow the instructions; they will show you the way. Spend twenty to thirty minutes a day or every other day learning and performing these exercises. In the beginning, have a simple goal of learning 1-3 stretches or exercises a day. The goal is to try all these exercises and if you don't feel comfortable with a particular stretch or exercise put it on the back burner and come back to it at a later date. You may surprise yourself when you return to it later. If you want to start with just one of the five books, that is ok. Pick up the others as you progress. They are all great! Remember to use your local library.

Why should we exercise? For good health and to feel better. We want to lift your mood through exercise creating good vibrations. I hope you will follow me on this path, the good path, the one less traveled. I have taken a smorgasbord of exercises that I feel you absolutely positively need to perform and divided them into 30-minute sessions you can perform once a day or once every other day until the path is completed.

Triangle Training --The Power of the Pyramid – The Program

10-minute warm-up stretch, 10-minute strength exercise, 10-minute warm-down stretch, a perfect triangle, as easy as 1,2,3.

The workout is like a good story; it has a beginning, a middle, and an end. First, we will warm up for ten minutes with a few stretching exercises. Next, we will do one strength exercise for ten minutes. For the strength exercise, we will do 3 sets of 15 repetitions, or 5 sets of 9, or 9 sets of 5 for a total of 45 reps in ten minutes or less. And finally, we will warm down by stretching again for the final 10 minutes. Sounds simple? Strength is important but we will spend twice as much time on flexibility and balance at FeelingGoodYou. The difference between a young athlete and an older athlete is flexibility and balance. **Being flexible and maintaining good balance is, in many ways, the fountain of youth**!

Stretching, Flexibility, Balance, Breathing and Water 101

There are different ways to stretch and I'm going to introduce a few stretching modalities to help the beginning stretcher. But first, let's start with breathing for stretching.

Breathing for Stretching

The five books all have a slightly different way of explaining how to breathe. To keep it simple let's just say the goal is to always breathe through your nose in and out. Assuming you are new to stretching, breathing through your nose may be difficult to do, and in some of the different stretches, e.g., standing on your head, it will be more difficult. As a rule of thumb breathe thru your nose when you can, otherwise breathe thru your mouth. Try to relax and keep the air flowing slowly and smoothly, and as you advance strive to take deeper more relaxed breaths.

Some stretches or asanas will be strenuous. If you start breathing too heavily, slow down.

There are many tricky breathing techniques in yoga and the yogis will tell you not to mess with most of them until after a year or so of yoga. As you advance you can work on the Darth Vader breath. When I make the Ha sound (in & out) while stretching, I feel like a yogi.

An Introduction to Stretching

To get started with stretching or Yoga you might want to start with the 12 posture Sun Salute, which is a small yoga circuit. Some people say the Sun Salutation is 5000 years old, others say it's only a hundred years old? Whatever the truth is, I do find a little magic in the Sun Salute and I hope you will find it too! To perform this circuit, you can check out my Free Guide https://access.feelinggoodyou.com/free. It will show you easy step-by-step instructions and diagrams to help you follow along. Memorize the circuit and you will have a great, first-rate way to stretch for the rest of your life!

Another style of stretching is from the book by Bob Cooley called *The Genius of Flexibility*. He begins with a beginner routine called Energy Series 1 and claims that this series opens up meridians in the body, and that after doing these 16 stretches you will feel energized and euphoric. I agree with the author, and it is one of my favorite regimens because it is simple and it works. Mr. Cooley digs deep into the science behind his method. I encourage you to read it. Energy Series 1 is a good place to start for the beginner. Energy series 2 is intermediate, and Energy Series 4 gets a little challenging and can really get your heart rate going. Energy Series 3 is partner-assisted stretching, which is wonderful if you have a partner? You can mix and match a few exercises, but in a nutshell, this book is a great foundation for strength and flexibility. This style of stretching is a little different from the stretching we are typically used to where you hold a stretch for some time and then release. Instead, you will be performing repetitions similar to the push-up or sit-up. He also asks you to focus on contracting the muscles while stretching. Keep your repetitions to 6 at first and increase the repetitions to fit your level of fitness. There are 16 different stretches in each series. Over time, experiment with the more advanced series. Pick and choose your favorite exercises, or make your own

16 exercise series if you like? It's a great book of stretching and strength exercises, and Energy Series 1 is a great warm-up before any athletic event. Monitor your heart rate as you get into the advanced series.

Yoga

Yoga is a force to be reckoned with. I've always struggled with Yoga. With my accident, a lot of my body atrophied and froze up. I found Yoga to be very foreign, painful, and embarrassing, especially in a group. I had to practice at home because I was so pathetic. Yoga can make a big difference in your life or your athletic performance. The history of Yoga may go back 10,000 years, so the origin of Yoga is a little uncertain. If someone told me it was a gift from the Gods… I'd believe it.

One of the most respected yoga teachers or gurus in western culture that I am aware of is B.K.S. Iyengar. The book I recommend is *Yoga The Iyengar Way*, by Silva, Mira & Shyam Mehta. There are 8 series in this book, each series having between eight and eighteen different asanas or stretches and balances.

Hold the stretches while breathing through your nose. Stretching might be a little uncomfortable in the beginning; however, don't give up. In time the pain will disappear. No need to rush getting into the advanced positions. In the beginning, try to hold your stretches for approximately 15-30 seconds; advance gradually and comfortably to one minute. When you start going beyond this level the student has become the teacher.

Ballet

Our next regimen is *The New York City Ballet Workout*. These exercises may not all be defined as stretching, but they will help work on your strength, balance, coordination, and posture. Use these routines in place of yoga or stretching when you would like to. Ballet is very therapeutic. And when you start getting the hang of it you may just say to yourself, "this is way too beautiful."

Pilates

To keep it simple I have reserved a day or two to complete the Pilates workout in and of itself. It's a great workout and will take a little time to get familiar with the exercises and some effort to get through this workout. It's a lot of work, but it's worth it!

Water 101

Exercise near a convenient shower. Ice, hot water, steam, cold water, baths, all of these forms of water have amazing healing properties. Many religious followers get baptized in water. The Hindus get washed in the Ganges River for a spiritual awakening. Muslims shower before prayer. It's no secret that a shower makes you feel good and refreshed! You can use a shower as a good warm up and a cool down.

To get five stars at the end of your shower, turn the hot water off, and take a cold shower or a Scottish shower for 30 seconds. You will notice a change in your spirit as soon as you step out of the shower. After the shower put on some skin lotion. When you apply the skin lotion you are not only promoting and maintaining healthy skin, but you are covering your body with the Chi energy! Your body will be loose and ready to go. It's important to shower immediately after your exercise to feel your best! Alone a shower makes us feel good, but after even a light sweat it makes us feel all the better. Remember after every exercise session to jump in the shower, and get 5 stars! It's good for your body and mind!

The Heart of the Matter

Before we get started on the first day, we have to do a little math and calculating to find our target heart rate. Although it's a simple formula, make sure you go over it a few times and calculate the correct answer. You are allowed to cheat here. Grab a calculator or call a friend who's good at math :) The point is you need to figure out your target heart rate and get it right to get the most out of this program and feel your best from the very beginning. If you are not into math, you can use a heart monitor and exercise at a moderate pace; or you can exercise by a feeling of exertion which I would define as light. To hone in on the ideal pace for your exercise there is the Karvonen formula which we will describe in detail. We will also dive a little deeper and reveal other methods to reach your optimum level of exertion during exercise.

The Karvonen formula is used by NSCA personal trainers to determine your target heart rate. The Free Guide will help simplify the Karvonen Formula: https://access.feelinggoodyou.com/free.

The Karvonen Formula is:
Target Heart Rate = [(max HR – resting HR) x %Intensity] + resting HR

1. (MHR) Maximum Heart Rate = 220 – your age

2. (RHR) Resting Heart Rate is your heart rate while you are resting.

3. (HRR) Heart Rate Reserve = Maximum Heart Rate – Resting Heart rate

To get your resting heart rate, put your two fingers up next to your Adam's apple and count how many pulses you have in 60 seconds while resting. The amount of heartbeats per minute is referred to as bpm (beats per minute).

Once you have your heart rate reserve you can calculate your training heart rate:

Multiply your HRR by your preferred target heart rate (we are using an 85% target heart rate in example 4, and a 50% target heart rate in example 5).

4. (.85 x HRR) + RHR = Upper end of the training zone.

5. (.50 x HRR) + RHR = Lower end of the training zone. **This lower end 50% target heart rate is the zone we are interested in and will use for the entirety of this program.**

To think about this formula and its terminology, you have a Maximum Heart Rate for your age which is theoretically the maximum rate your heart can beat per minute. And you have a Resting Heart Rate which is your heart beats per minute while at rest. Your Target Heart Rate is somewhere between these two numbers. Your Heart Rate Reserve is the difference between these two numbers; your Maximum Heart Rate minus your Resting Heart Rate. To get your Target Heart Rate, multiply your Heart Rate Reserve by your preferred rate, which will be 50% or .50 in our case. Then simply add the Resting Heart Rate. After you calculate your Target Heart Rate per minute you will need to find out what your Target Heart Rate is for 15 seconds. Waiting a full minute to count your pulse is a little inconvenient, and loses accuracy as your pulse slows down significantly during the full minute. So, it's more efficient to determine your pulse in 15 seconds. To find this number simply divide your Target Heart Rate per minute by 4. This will give you a number you can easily access during your routine. So, go ahead and do the calculations and write that number down on your index card please, because we will be exercising shortly! Class dismissed.

Reaching this target heart rate is a big part of this program, or if you will the **heart of the program**. By reaching this target heart rate I believe our body triggers the feel-good endorphins which is why we can call it Supercalifragilistic, great, pure, righteous, high soaring spirits! And it is our objective to reach or get close to this target rate at least once during our 30-minute sessions. The strength exercises should make it easy to get to this rate in 1-2 minutes. In some workouts, we may reach the target 3 times or more, but typically when we reach our target heart rate, we will take a minute or so to rest and either sit or stand idly by, or spend our resting time doing a stretch until we recover.

You can purchase a heart monitor and many people prefer them, but from my experience taking your pulse the old-fashioned way is more accurate. In the beginning, take your pulse by hand or fingertips. After a week or so you will know your target heart rate by your breath and your feeling of exertion. A few months down the road, you can consider purchasing a heart monitor that will be able to put your workouts on a graph right on your smartphone or computer. You will gain insights into your workouts by quickly observing these graphs, and seeing at a glance which exercises spike your heart rate the most.

When you are performing a vigorous exercise take note of how you feel when you hit the 50% exertion rate. Pay attention to your breath and how heavy you are breathing through your nose. Your nose will tell you your optimum training level. Follow your nose. When you are not able to breathe through your nose anymore during exercise and need to breathe through your mouth to get more oxygen, you're going beyond your optimum training level.

How you feel after your workout is also important. Maybe you could have pushed a little harder, maybe you should have backed off a bit. You will figure this out in time, but for the time being, you are right where you need to be.

Climbing the Mountain

In order to stay forever young we should "keep moving". It's not my intention to overwhelm the reader with an abundance of exercises. I want to show people that there are many different ways up the mountain. And by trying different exercises you can discover what exercises you enjoy the most, and add a little variety to your routine while exercising different muscles. You will also find your favorite way of catching the feeling good you flow.

In the beginning I'd like you to focus on your pace. Imagine yourself in the back of the pack. The exercise pace I recommend is a 50% exertion rate which is considerably lower than what most personal trainers would recommend, upward around 70-85% (Rocky 100%). At first you may feel unsatisfied with the workout; and get a feeling that you're not pushing hard enough. Just hang in there for a few workouts, pay attention to your breath, your heart rate, and your overall feeling of exertion. Subscribe to my Free Guide that has illustrated instructions, and teaches you step by step how to catch the exercise high. I show you here in the book too, but I think the pictures in the guide are helpful. I want you to focus on feeling good while performing the simplest of exercises.

One of the beautiful things about strength training is its ability to quickly get your heart rate up to your target heart rate. If you're new to strength training I suggest you start with a few push ups. This is a wonderful strength exercise that requires no equipment, and gives you the ability to reach your target heart rate in approximately 1 minute, even if you are doing push ups on your knees. By doing push ups we can easily catch the exercise high. If you are beginning you may want to stick to this one exercise until you are comfortable with the routine. I will demonstrate the entire framework in the guide. In the guide, I recommend a modified deadlift exercise to get you started which is also very basic. Maybe you have a sore elbow, and can't do push ups. All you really need is one strength exercise to effortlessly catch the exercise high.

The next simple strength exercise to work on would be the sit-up. It may take a little longer to get your heart rate up, but this is a good foundational exercise. Personally I like to cheat a little while doing sit-ups, and I'll use my arms to swing, gaining a little momentum and then I'll touch my toes with my fingers.

The pull-up, although well known, is a fairly advanced exercise. Maybe that's why the pull-up bars in the parks always seem so lonely? So, if you're slowly moving up the mountain the next step after the sit-ups may be to purchase a 5lb. kettlebell, and work on your deadlifts and kettlebell swings. This is an easy and seemingly effortless way to increase your heart rate. You can work on catching the exercise high and feeling good at your own pace, but be consistent.

While climbing the mountain we will be doing different exercises, but our objective is always to feel good. After you start learning to feel good with several different exercises you will become a master at catching the exercise high, and you will be able to change your mood at will! With time and persistence you will learn the art of catching the exercise high!!!

One thing I loved about the martial arts was that in some ways it made me a worldly person. Maybe I haven't traveled around the world, but through martial arts I have met people from all over the world: Brazil, Columbia, Venezuela, South Korea, Israel, Africa, Czechoslovakia, Cambodia, Sweden, Japan, China, Russia, Philippines, really anywhere and everywhere. So with that in mind I have included exercise routines and exercises from all around the globe. When designing this program I did take into consideration that not only did I want to have exercises for people with different capabilities, but I wanted to show people exercises that originated from all over the world. Qigong for example originated in the Tibetan Mountains of South Asia, and it can be a very stress free form of exercise with modifications for people that are handicapped. Capoeira is more advanced, and has its roots in Africa, and Brazil. Pilates has its roots in Germany, and the United States. Ballet traces its roots to the Italian Renaissance. I hope you can search and find your favorite routine while climbing the mountain!!! To your health!

If you have a question or feel overwhelmed you can contact me at info@ jimringers.com for a free consultation.

I love exercise and I use exercise to improve my mood, and increase my energy effortlessly. This is what I want for you, and this is my reason for writing this book.

Strongman Exercises: Getting Strong Now

The Eight Great Strength Exercises:

- The Push-up
- The Sit-up
- The Pull-up
- The Squat
- The Deadlift
- Kettlebell Swings and Snatches
- The Bridge
- The Turkish Get-up

The advantage of high-intensity workouts, e.g., strength exercises, is they will increase your metabolism, help you lose weight, feel great, build muscle and increase strength. However, we are going to modify a typical weight lifting workout by controlling our heart rate. We will do this by monitoring our pulse and taking a rest when we reach our target heart rate.

By training at this low end or 50% exertion rate, there will be very little discomfort in our exercise. Another big advantage is your form and performance will be significantly better. Contrary to popular opinion, when it comes to weightlifting you don't need to put your body under the stress of maximum repetitions. You may not gain the strength and muscle size of a competitive weight lifter, but you will keep your body strong, and significantly reduce the chances of injury. Simply monitor your heart rate and when you reach your target heart rate take a break and rest or stretch for approximately one minute, or as short as ten seconds, or until you feel good? In this program, you will not be grimacing and straining to finish your last repetition. It's an easier, less stressful, and arguably more effective way to train. More enjoyable for sure.

Supercalifragilistic Time

Grab your index card with your target heart rate. Or just memorize your target heart rate for 15 seconds because we will be using it shortly.

Day 1. The 30-minute Workout with 45 Push-Ups

Step 1: The 10-minute warm-up

If you like you can spend the first 10 minutes learning and trying to memorize the Sun Salutation circuit. You can find the circuit in my Free Guide or in the book *Body, Mind, and Sport*. Perform 5-10 circuits. One circuit should be approximately 1 minute. Breathe deep at every transition. Or you can start with Bob Cooley's Energy Series 1, for ten minutes?

To keep it simple, swing a baseball bat, or a golf club nice and easy for ten minutes. This simple little exercise is a full-body exercise and will warm you up from the tips of your toes to your fingertips.

Step 2: 45 Push-ups in 10 minutes

After the 10-minute warm-up, perform 45 push-ups while taking breaks between sets. Since it is our first day, you can start with 9 sets of 5 reps. for the push-ups. You have 10 minutes to perform 45 push-ups without going over your target heart rate. Take a break during your sets to monitor your heart rate. Start with 5 push-ups, regular ones or on your knees. Finish your first set, monitor your heart rate, and check to see your pulse is at or below the 50% exertion level. It may take a few sets before you reach your target heart rate, but begin to take note of how you feel and breathe at that exertion point.

While you are waiting for your heart rate to come down do a couple of easy stretches, or just sit American Indian style as you recover. You can also sit on the mat, grab your knees, and rock back and forth. That is a good way to recover between the strength exercises! Let your pulse come down, and get ready for your next set. When your breathing is relaxed you are ready to continue. Repeat the procedure monitoring your pulse throughout the rest of your push-ups, and taking a break when you reach your target heart rate.

Congratulations, you did 45 push-ups! It should make you feel good. If you are unable to complete 45 push-ups in the allotted 10 minutes that's fine too; write down the number you did complete on the index card and move on to the stretching. If by chance you are in good shape, and while doing the push-ups you never reached your target heart rate, do as many push-ups as it takes to reach the target heart rate in the allotted 10 minutes.

Step 3: The 10-minute warm-down
Spend the remaining time stretching. A good place to start is with the Sun Salutation circuit. Repeat the circuit daily until you memorize it. When you get bored, move on to Energy Series 1 in Bob Cooley's book. Repeat that series until you memorize it. These two series alone should be enough to get you through the first few weeks. Take your time studying the stretches. You can apply the studying time and reading time to the ten minutes warm-up and warm-down (or cool down?). If you feel more comfortable just swinging a baseball bat at first that's ok too, it's a good stretch.

After 30 minutes total, you have finished the exercises. Congratulations!

Don't forget to jump in the shower, and get 5 stars!
Be cognizant of the way you feel after the workout, and for the rest of the day. You should feel good. It's important to feel good, that is what makes you want to come back and do it again tomorrow or the next day.

Day 2. The Sit-Up
Step 1: The 10-minute warm-up
Start with a warm-up of stretching for ten minutes. If you are new to stretching you will need to get accustomed to breaking down the stretches in these books. Look at the pictures and read what the author has written by the stretch to make things easier. Don't worry about doing the perfect stretch; just do the best you can. And relax and take it easy as opposed to forcing yourself and pushing beyond your limits. The process will take time, but for now, it's only ten minutes. Enjoy the journey!

Step 2: 45 sit-ups
Begin the sit-ups by anchoring your feet with something. A ten-pound dumbbell or kettlebell on one foot works fine. Place your foot through the kettlebell handle. Alternate the foot after each set. After some time, you will strengthen your muscles and will not need to anchor your feet.

Repeat the same procedure as we did for the push-ups. Do a set and take a rest. Monitor your pulse and keep your heart rate at or below the 50% exertion level. Keep going until you complete the 45 reps. or until the ten minutes have expired.

Step 3: The 10-minute warm-down
Stretch for ten minutes or the remaining time. It's perfectly fine to stick with the Sun Salutation and Energy Series 1 for the first month or two. When you feel like advancing and trying new stretches you have plenty of material. Whether it's Energy Series 2 and 4 in Bob Cooley's Genius of Flexibility, or from any of the material in the yoga or ballet books. Take your time, and you'll know when you're ready to advance.

Day 3. The Pull-Up
Step 1: The 10-minute warm-up
Start with a 10-minute stretching warm-up. I still prefer to warm up by swinging the Indian Club or baseball bat. Spend part of the ten minutes learning a new stretch as well.

Step 2: 45 pull-ups

Pull-ups are strenuous so keep an eye on your pulse. Rest and breathe a bit to keep your heart rate at or below the 50% exertion rate.

If you struggle with pull-ups try performing a negative pull-up instead. Jump up so your chin is over the bar. Slowly go down counting to 5, a thousand one, a thousand two, etc. Perform a set of negative pull-ups. Rest between sets, and monitor your pulse until you do 45 total, or until the ten minutes is up.

If that is too difficult, try to just hang from the pull-up bar for 15-30 seconds or longer. Try that a few times. After 10 minutes, move on to the stretch.

Step 3: The 10-minute warm-down

Spend 10 minutes stretching for your warm down. If you are holding your stretches, 30 seconds is a good number to shoot for at all levels.

Day 4. The Deadlift
Step 1: The 10-minute warm-up

Start with a ten-minute stretching warm-up. Sometimes it's nice to use a stretching assistant like those exercise bands. A belt or even a t-shirt will work too.

Step 2: 45 deadlifts

A good way to practice the deadlift is to get in the football stance. Get one hand on the floor as if you were a running back or a lineman for a football team. If your right hand is on the mat, your left forearm should be resting above your left knee. Now stand up, and switch. Now left hand on the mat, right forearm resting above your right knee. Now stand up, and switch. Do that 15 times each side, or do as many as it takes to get to your target heart rate, or until your ten minutes has expired.

If you have the ten lb. kettlebell, start with it. Grab the kettlebell with both hands similar to a running back, except both hands are grabbing the kettlebell; keep your chin slightly up and lift the weight off the floor, rock back a little like a weeble-wobble and push through your heels, come all the way up. Now go back down to the mat. Repeat the deadlift a total of 45 times, resting and monitoring your pulse between sets. Nine sets of five repetitions is a good place to start.

If you need extra help with this exercise, search for videos on the deadlift on YouTube and watch an instructional or two. Take your time moving up in weight, and keep a close eye on your heart rate.

Step 3: The 10-minute warm-down
Stretch 10 minutes for your warm down. It will take a while for most people to breathe through their noses while stretching. Keep working on it, if you are a big spender think about purchasing those breathe-right strips. They will give you some help.

Day 5. Pilates
The Pilates workout is situated right in the middle of the strength exercises just to mix it up a bit. Follow *The Pilates Powerhouse*, by Mari Winsor to the best of your ability for 30 minutes. You might want to do half the exercises one day and the other half the following day. You will not need to stretch or do a strength exercise with the Pilates workout; as there is a lot of yoga, flexibility and strength incorporated into the workout already. However, if you would prefer to use the triangle training choose your favorite strength exercise, and feel free to mix it into the middle of the workout.

This is a challenging series so take your time learning the exercises and routines. Eventually, you will be strong enough to make it through the whole series in one day. You will feel good!

Day 6. The Assisted Squat
Step 1: The 10-minute warm-up
Ease into a 10-minute stretching warm-up. Dynamic stretching is preferred by most experts to begin your workout. Swinging the bat, The Genius of Flexibility, Pilates, Qigong, balletic plie exercises, and the Sun Salute

are all examples of dynamic stretching or using movement to stretch your muscles.

Step 2: 45 squats

To perform the assisted squat, find a railing, a banister, a table, or a dance bar, something that comes up to a height around your belly button. Let's say you have a railing like this on your deck. Grab the railing with both hands (watch for splinters; wear gloves), square the feet to the railing, and then point your toes out a wee bit at about shoulder-width apart. Lean back, and bend your knees, to a squatting position so that your knees are at a 90-degree angle (or a little lower if you are a risk-taker). Use your arms and legs to pull yourself back to the standing position; similar to a wakeboarder coming out of the water. Do 3 sets of 15 or whatever combination works best for you for a total of 45 assisted squats. To increase the intensity, try performing this exercise with only one hand. If you start breathing heavily, check your pulse and keep at or below the target heart rate.

As you progress you can look into the different types of squats. There is the front squat, the back squat, and the goblet squat, just to name a few. While the squat exercise is very effective in general, it's also very advanced, and you would be wise to proceed with caution. Use light weight and focus on good form.

Step 3: The 10-minute warm-down

A 10-minute warm down. Static stretching is when you hold your stretch, preferably for up to 30 seconds. Many people prefer static stretching at the end of a workout. Yoga has many different static stretching positions.

While holding your stretch you might prefer to try this breathing routine:

1. Breathe out, through your nose for seven seconds.
2. Breathe in, through your nose for seven seconds.
3. Hold your breath for one second.
4. Repeat approximately 2-4 times, while holding your stretch.

I prefer to use a metronome or clock when any counting is involved. Otherwise, I tend to speed up the count.

Day 7. Turkish Get-Ups
Step 1: The 10-minute warm-up
Warm-up stretch for 10 minutes. Try 5 minutes of the Sun Salute, and 5 minutes of *The Genius of Flexibility.*

Step 2: 10 Turkish Get-Ups on each side
The Turkish get-up is a sit-up and a lunge combined. We will start with a sixteen-ounce bottle of water as our weight. **This is an advanced exercise. If you don't feel comfortable with this exercise, you can skip it for now.** You might go on YouTube and check out a couple of videos for this one. It's a lot easier to watch a video than to read about the intricacies of this exercise, but I will give you a written explanation here:

Sit on the mat with your feet out in front, grab the sixteen-ounce water bottle with your left hand and lift it over your head (keep holding it above your head until you lie down at the end). Place your left foot on the mat by your right knee. Post your right hand on the mat by your right hip. Bring your right foot back through your right hand and your posted left foot. Imagine your right leg is the arrow on a bow and arrow, and you are drawing it back through your posted left foot and right hand. After drawing it back through the bow, post it up on your right knee. Swivel your right foot to the right where you are now in a lunge position. Use your toes to perform an upward lunge and stand up into a standing position holding the water bottle above your head the whole time…going down now…step back with the right foot. Put your right knee down on the mat. Swivel the foot. Kick the right foot back through the bow. Use your stomach muscles to lie down on the mat. Now, do the left side.

You can start with five or ten reps on each side and gradually work your way up to ten or fifteen reps on each side. Whatever you can comfortably do in ten minutes. Check your pulse and relax as much as possible. Feeling good is good enough. This is an advanced exercise, but I believe in exercises that help you get off the floor and into a standing position. It develops real natural strength.

Step 3: The 10-minute warm-down
Cool down for 10 minutes. Try 5 minutes of the Sun Salute, and 5 minutes of yoga?

Day 8. Kettlebell Swings and Snatches
Step 1: The 10-minute warm-up
Do a warm-up stretch for 10 minutes. Hopefully, you have figured out the sun-salutation by now? If not, keep looking at the diagrams.

Step 2: 45 kettlebell swings
A kettlebell swing is pretty simple. Watch a video or two on this one too. Begin with a shoulder-width stance or just a bit wider. Grab the kettlebell, with two hands, and swing the 10-pound kettlebell between your legs with both hands. If you don't have a kettlebell, you can do the swing with no weight or an imaginary kettlebell or just grab your 16-ounce water bottle, or your preferred weight. Swing the weight up to head height and swing it back down between your knees. Perform 45 kettlebell swings, and rest, when necessary.

If you have extra time, you can also perform the snatch exercise for a set of 15. Start in a standing position with your feet shoulder-width apart, and a kettlebell on the floor between your big toes. Bend over and grab the kettlebell with both hands. Lean back slightly and swing the kettlebell above your head and feel the power going through your heels. Slowly and comfortably bring the kettlebell back down to the mat. Repeat.

As you advance you can begin to experiment with the one-handed kettlebell swings. Take precautions not to drop the kettlebell especially if you live in an upstairs apartment! You will also discover that you can do upwards of 150 kettlebell swings in the allotted ten minutes, so no need to race to get there. If you decide to purchase a heavier kettlebell, move up in weight slowly. The kettlebell is a great way to get your heart rate up quickly and easily so keep an eye on your target heart rate. It's more conservative and easier on your joints to reach the target rate in two minutes with a ten-pound weight as opposed to increasing the weight and reaching the target heart rate in only one minute.

Step 3: The 10-minute warm-down

Stretch for 10 minutes. If you have been working on energy series one, see how many exercises you can get through in ten minutes. Keep the repetitions to six at first.

Have a great day!

Day 9. Bridges
45 Bridges to warm up

The Hip Bridge—15 reps.

Lie down on the mat with hands by your side. With your feet on the mat, lift your hips up. Bring your hips back down to the floor, do 15 repetitions.

Beginners do 3 sets of hip bridges.

(The following exercise is advanced; proceed with caution and make sure you are comfortable performing a headstand before you attempt this exercise.)

Assisted Neck Bridge for 15 reps. (1-3 sets) … getting warmer:

Start with your back on the mat, hands by your head, and lift your hips up. With the palms of your hands on the mat, inverted, next to your ear, rock your head backward and bring your hips up, and back down to the floor. Repeat 15 times.

Regular Bridge (1-3 sets) … climbing the mountain:

Do the regular bridge, for 15 repetitions. Lift your hips up and with the palms of your hands next to your head, lift your head off the floor and make the bridge as high as you can. Can you bridge on your tippy-toes? It took me a while. Then bring your head and hips back down to the floor. Repeat 15 times. Check your pulse here, this is a vigorous exercise!

It took some time, but after I became accustomed to getting into the Buddha or Lotus position; I would do that at this moment to rest between sets. Here, I feel on top of the mountain!

Stationary Bridge (1-3 sets)
Do one bridge and hold. Lift your head off the mat, and hold it for 15 breaths. If possible, breathe through your nose. When I say this is a vigorous exercise, I mean it is easy to get your heart beating rapidly. To keep your heart at a moderate rate; you may need to stop and rest or slow down your exercise.

Bridge on a wall, cooling down.
Find a wall and lean backward to the wall placing your palms against the wall. Walk your hands down the wall until you feel a good stretch. Then walk your hands back up the wall, and repeat 7 times.

I consider all the bridges, strength, and stretch exercises, so you don't have to stretch afterward…unless you are up for extra credit or points and stars? After 30 minutes you're done!

Day 10. The Ballet Workout
Spend 30 minutes with *The New York City Ballet Workout.*

Have fun! In time you will be sophisticated and part of the aristocracy. :)

Or, do the triangle training?

Step 1: Warm-up with 10 minutes of *The NYC Ballet Workout*

Step 2. Strength or Cardio
Perform your favorite strength or cardio exercise for ten minutes, if you wish?

Step 3: Warm down with 10 minutes of *The NYC Ballet Workout*

Ballet makes me feel like a tree dancing in the wind. When I started performing ballet exercises, specifically the Ballet Center exercises in the back of the book, I felt like I had no roots, and the slightest breeze would have me topple over. As time passed, my roots began to grow as if they were growing from my feet into the floor and eventually deep into the earth. Because of my accident, I'm still a little unstable on my feet, but the improvement has been dramatic. Studies show that as we get older losing our balance, and taking a fall can be all too common and often lead to our demise. It's important to work on our ballet. If you are a macho man, do a little shadow boxing between sets. Don't forget to listen to sophisticated music, and remember, someone has to be the Prima Donna.

Day 11. Jump Rope and Run

Step 1: The 10-minute warm-up

Warm-up for 10 minutes. You may want to warm up with 10 minutes of the assisted squat if you see a railing nearby?

Step 2: Jump Rope

Find the right type of platform to jump rope: a tennis court, a basketball court, or a wooden platform. It may help to have a 5' by 5' rug to throw down on the surface to add some extra cushion. Be careful, although you probably jumped rope as a kid, this **is an advanced exercise.** If you feel uncomfortable jumping rope, substitute a walk or jog for 10 minutes. If you think you are up for it, start slowly. Begin with ten jump ropes, and see how you feel? Gradually move up to 100-300 jump ropes, 10-50 at a time, taking breaks between sets, and monitoring your heart! Jumping rope is another fabulous exercise and a great way to get your heart pounding. Unfortunately, the risk for your knees, ankles, and hips, is also elevated a tad, so use good judgment. Pace yourself, monitor your heart rate, and rest between sets with breaths through your nose. Stretch while resting between sets, any stretch will do, touch your toes, do a calf stretch, maybe a sun salutation, or maybe look up to the sky and watch an eagle fly?

Step 3: 45-yard runs

When you start to run, be very careful and start slowly. It can be very easy to pull and strain muscles when you begin the 45-yard runs. Monitor your heart rate and keep it at or below 50%. Take it easy, and slowly, over time, increase your volume. Step up to the starting line and simply run for 45 yds. Start with 3-5 45-yard runs and work your way up to about 8 45-yard runs. Concentrate on your form. When you feel you were **born to run,** then you know you are on the right track!

Stretch between runs, take plenty of extra breaths to recover. Rest at both ends with deep breaths preferably through your nose.

More Advanced

On the way back to the original starting line, run 45 yards backward at a very relaxed pace.

After your second run, do 15 high steps for each leg back to the starting line between runs. A high step is similar to punting a football; hold your hand out front and try to kick your hand. Do 15 reps. with each leg.

After your third run, go back to the start running sideways at a relaxed pace, head to the east.

After your fourth run, go back to the start running sideways at a relaxed pace, facing the west.

If you prefer, you can split these two workouts up and follow the same basic model: warming up for ten minutes, doing the exercise (running or jump rope), and then cooling down for ten minutes. But since they both take you outside, I like to do them together, and simply stretch between exercises. Both these exercises will easily get you up to your target zone, so better to take it easy and slow. Strive to perform the 45-yard runs with great form. And relax with the jump ropes, start with low reps and long breaks.

No need to warm down, we have been stretching between sets, maybe a short walk?

Hit the showers!

Day 12. Hula Hooping and Qigong
Saving the best for last,

To begin Qigong simply surf the internet and you will find all kinds of introductory courses for free. You can simply follow along, or pick up a copy of *The Qigong Bible*, by Katherine Allen. Qigong has thousands of exercises so opening this book is almost like entering another dimension. Qigong will teach you how to relax and go with the flow!

Qigong is also our go-to exercise if you find some of the exercises in this program too advanced. Qigong is great for senior citizens and has modified movements for people with disabilities. Qigong is truly a beautiful art for the people of this world.

Step 1: Warm-up with 10 minutes of Qigong

Step 2: Hula Hoop for 10 minutes
If you have never Hula Hooped before you are missing out! It is a great way to get your heart rate up in about 2 minutes. If you want to learn how to Hula Hoop get yourself one of those Hula Hoops with ridges inside. Work on doing about 45 Hula Hoops, then take a rest. Do 45 more in the opposite direction, take a rest. Once you get the hang of it you will be able to do 100-300 hulas at a time. While getting started rest and hula for equal time for ten minutes (1-minute hula, 1-minute rest). Have you ever heard the expression, "it's all in the hips."?

Step 3: Warm down with Qigong for 10 minutes
Or, for day 12 just try something else for 30 minutes? Try Tai Chi, riding a bike, rock climbing, hiking, surfing, dancing, skydiving, skating, gardening, shadow boxing, swing some Indian clubs, or a golf club. If you're young

and adventurous try a martial art or boxing, you get the idea. Day 12 is trying something new, or staying home with some Qigong?

Day 13. But wait there's more--the Swim.

I encourage you to read the book *Total Immersion*, by Terry Laughlin for swimming instruction.

Find yourself a local swimming pool. Take a swim lesson if necessary. We all know swimming is a great exercise, just do it! Any type of swimming for thirty minutes will suffice.

One of the pitfalls of this program is you will spend more time than you might like being cold and wet, LOL! Your negative self will do battle to talk you out of all the great benefits that are ahead of you both physically and mentally from the swim. As you head to the pool the negative forces will be in full power talking you out of your swim…the time, the inconvenience, the cold water. Anything it needs to do to stop you, you must carry on! For me, the swim is the battlefield of the mind. The swim can wash away disturbing emotions like hatred, anger, annoyance, aggravation, irritation, ill-temper, resentment, fear, bitterness, greed, dissatisfaction, revenge, greed, jealousy, ill will, befouled, indecent, obscene, and impure thoughts. And wash into the mind positive emotions and a feeling of joy, thanksgiving, faith, enthusiasm, hope, desire, and gratefulness. Demons can't swim. After a swim, you may see the beauty in this world?!

As you advance:
Do equal time for the breaststroke, backstroke, butterfly, and freestyle stroke. Start with 30-minute workouts, gradually working up to 45 minutes. While resting at the wall, practice breathing through your nose and doing the Darth Vader exhale, 15-40 breaths should have you on your way again. Rest to recover after each IM (IM is an individual medley or a swim competition involving all four strokes) or rest in between butterfly laps, or whenever you want to, typically the temperature of the water will be your motivating factor to get moving, LOL? If you can't do the butterfly, do the breaststroke, try one butterfly, maybe two? If you can eventually

do the butterfly for 25 yds., you're making big progress. Jack LaLanne referred to the butterfly as the greatest exercise. Rest assured it will have your spirit fly as well!

In all the other exercises I have instructed you to keep your heart rate at or under your 50% exertion rate. For the majority of the swim, I keep my heart rate in check, and I like to relax and take some deep recovery breaths on the wall. However, if I'm feeling good, I may race for 50-200 yds. towards the end of the swim? Talk about breaking the yoke and setting yourself free!

I don't do any extra strength or stretching on swim day. If you have the time and energy it's a good idea to stretch after the swim.

Day 14. Have a beer or a glass of wine. Enjoy a bath. Get some therapy.
Take an Epsom salt bath for 15-20 minutes, it helps to relieve aches and pains. Add some olive oil, coconut oil, and shea butter to your bath; it's good for your skin. You might want to go get a massage to work on some tight muscles. I also recommend *therapy balls* to work out some of the kinks. And finally, to relax, enjoy a beer or a glass of wine; some studies show an occasional beer or glass of wine is good for your heart. If you would prefer an herbal tea, remember it's your day, choose your favorite beverage!

After a few months and you see that your belt is a few notches tighter, maybe you should have a night on the town? Call your friends and tell them, "I'm feeling good and looking good." Break out a pair of fancy shoes and socks. Maybe a stylish hat? Walk beautifully, talk beautifully, live beautifully.

Day 15. Begin again.
You do not need to perform these workouts in the order presented. For example, on Day 2 you may decide to swim. You may like swimming and decide to swim three times a week. Stick to the basic plan and try to get all the workouts in within a 2-4-week period as a general guideline. If you would like to change the order of the workouts around for your

purposes that is fine. And if you have a problem with a particular exercise for some reason, and you decide to skip it, that is understandable. Do the best you can. On the other hand, if you are feeling good, and would like to carry your workouts over the 30-minute mark, or fit in two workouts a day, that's ok too; just remember to look, listen and feel and keep the workouts at or below the 50% target heart rate.

On the warm-ups and warm-downs keep in mind that you can warm up and down with ballet, qigong, yoga (Sun Salutation), Pilates, or the Genius of Flexibility exercises. You may want to find your own stretches or dance moves? You can spend more time on your favorite exercises, but if you are capable, it's also important to work on a little bit of everything in the two-week circuit. Don't get overwhelmed by the number of exercises in each platform. Do what you can do in 10-20 minutes and move on.

With the strength exercises, 45 reps is a good estimate for the number of reps you should get in for the allotted 10 minutes. All the exercises are a little different so things will vary. In the beginning, you may do a little less, and as you progress you may feel the need to do some more.

Remember to jump in the shower after every workout, and get 5 stars! It's good for your body and spirit!

Working Your Way Down the Path

Month 3

Start challenging yourself with more stretches. It's good to perform stretches and routines you are familiar with, but it is also important to keep branching out and discovering new stretches at your own pace. Teach yourself one to three new stretches or balances at a time, and before you know it, you will be familiar with hundreds of different stretches and balances.

As you progress you will eventually be able to perform the Lotus position. The Lotus position looks like the American Indian style position except your feet are crossed over one another. You will often see statues of famous far-east people like Buddha in some sort of Lotus position. This is a good meditation posture and a great position to rest and stretch in between high-intensity exercises or a perfect ending to any workout.

Work on your ballet stretches too and focus on the moves that require balance, poise, finesse, and gracefulness. If you are persistent you will notice steady improvement.

To make a homemade stretching tool take an old tennis racquet, and cut all the strings out of the racquet. Now you have a great assistant stretching tool. For starters you can hook the racquet around your foot, and do a toe touch. Hook it onto anything, and work more on your stretching. You can also use the de-stringed tennis racquet to swing like a baseball bat or any club really. This is good because the light weight can work better for different swings. Have fun!

Another little secret.

When you think about it, we have our whole world in our hands; laundry, grocery, shopping, yard work, computers, and if you like sports like tennis, golf, baseball, football, racquetball. A good grip is important especially to elite athletes. In martial arts, the fighting usually begins and ends with the hands. I believe the hands are your most valuable tool. Maybe it's the opposable thumb, but a good grip will help you in most sports. If you want results, find the time to work your hands. It takes less than ten minutes a day. **The Sidewinder** grip products helped to strengthen my hands. They have three products that I am aware of: The Grip Twister, the Pro Extreme, and the Revolution. I have the Grip Twister and the Pro Extreme. The Pro Extreme is my favorite. They are both fairly expensive (over $100?) so, you will have to make a sacrifice to get strong hands, but it's worth it. Start with 15 reps in all five directions and work your way up to 45 repetitions. You can substitute it for any strength exercise. You can work your hands almost every day; start with three times a week.

And another tool you can treat yourself to is a pair of 2-pound Indian Clubs. They are shaped like a bowling pin and you can use them for a great warm-up or warm-down exercise. You can use them for cardio exercises too. A good wake-up warm-up is simply swinging an Indian club like a baseball bat lefty and righty. And with a little imagination or an instructional tape, you can do countless exercises with these clubs! There are plenty of good simple exercise products out there; choose the one that you like the best, and it will be easy to plug right into this system.

Hey, man or woman, we are getting strong now. We are working our hands and our wrists and shoulders too! You will feel the difference in just a couple of weeks and will start to notice the difference when opening a twist-off coke or a jar of peanut butter; life is good. We are feeling good. We are looking good!

The Country Club

I would like to expand a little on using your Indian Club or Country Club (any club approximately 1-3 feet long) for an all-around complete workout. As I mentioned a few times, it's nice to warm up by swinging the Indian Club. For me, the Country Club or Indian Club is the best way to comfortably ease into your workout. And we can use a stick, a baseball bat, a tennis racquet, or a golf club to swing in its place even if we don't have an Indian Club handy. If we start by swinging our club like a baseball bat it will take approximately one minute to swing your club fifteen times. So, let's use fifteen repetitions for each exercise and it will be easy for us to plan and time our workouts. I like to call this routine my Country Club Routine because it prepares me for the country club. And hopefully, when you start feeling good and looking good you will get an invitation to the country club and these exercises will help you prepare for the activities at hand.

The baseball swing:

The baseball swing is just what it sounds like. Swing your Indian Club, stick, or bat like a baseball bat for two minutes, one minute on each side. After just two minutes you will already start feeling loose as a goose. You will feel more alive and prepared for your workout.

Swing number two: Step into your swing and bring your back foot past your front foot. If you wish, at the end of the swing look back towards your bat and feel the stretch, turn your head the opposite way too for another light stretch. You will be twisting your spine, so as with all of your stretches feel the stretch, but take it easy.

Swing number three: Now, instead of crossing your feet take the front foot and point your toes approximately 90 degrees forward. If you are familiar with yoga, the feet are in the Warrior Pose position, the back foot pointing east and the front foot pointing north. Step forward a few inches if it feels comfortable, and lightly swing the bat. Look ahead and feel the stretch.

The tennis swing:

Now we are beginning to prepare you for the country club. To start with, use your club or a tennis racquet and perform a simple forehand shot. Follow with the backhand shot for fifteen repetitions. You should feel this working on your shoulders and wrists. It will also work your legs and hips as you shift your weight from side to side. It is a good idea to start with a lightweight stick or a tennis racquet for this exercise.

With these few exercises, we have already completed our normal ten-minute warm-up. The following exercises you can perform as you see fit.

The tennis serve:

Throw an imaginary ball up in the air and slowly follow through with your stick or racquet past your opposite foot. I also refer to this movement as the baseball pitch because it is similar to it but without throwing the imaginary ball up in the air.

The golf swing:

Hey, let me tell you something, golf isn't that easy. And it takes practice, but performing the basic golf swing with the Country Club is a good start. This will build all the muscles you need to lift the golf club, follow-through, and hit the ball! And you can practice indoors without having to worry about busting a few lamps or TVs. Don't underestimate the value of this swing. If you like golf, perform this swing for approximately five minutes. This motion and repetition will transfer to the golf course and help your game.

To increase your heart rate for the second part of the workout, swing the club like a kettlebell or an ax chopping wood, or just swing the club in any direction a little faster. Your arms may feel a little fatigued after this vigorous part of the workout? Use the club to perform a couple basic stretches to cool down. Hold it behind your feet for a little stretch, or above your head for a backbend and maybe to the side? Finish off with a few light swings.

Using the Country Club will prepare you for the country club. Once you start feeling good and looking good the world will become your oyster. Don't worry about being club champion, just practice enough to avoid embarrassing yourself. Get out and socialize with the one-percenters, it beats caddying. Enjoy the rolling hills, walking through nature, and breathing the fresh air. You should feel a bit more… civilized?

The soccer ball

And then there was soccer or futbol? I know it's a little confusing, but soccer is the world's largest sport, isn't it?

To follow the regular triangle training, you can kick the ball around lightly for 10 minutes. Then pick up the pace a bit by jogging a little behind the ball, and reaching your target heart rate for the following ten minutes. And finally, relax a bit with a light walk and a few extra kicks for the last ten minutes. That's your basic soccer feelinggoodyou workout.

Here are a few more ideas:

You might want to deflate the ball a bit. That way, it doesn't move so fast. Try kicking it against a wall. Fifteen kicks with both feet is a good start.

Try that a few times… getting bored?

Throw in a couple of cartwheels or handstands in, if you can? Maybe a headstand or a frog stand? Kick your soccer ball around the soccer field, jog a little as you dribble, throw in a few extra kicks. Kick your soccer ball home for ten minutes. Kicking the soccer ball makes you feel more… international?

Going Lefty

It's important and rewarding to work on your opposite side. In a way, it's kind of sad how many people have put their left hand or right hand and, for that matter, foot "on the bench"—so to say. If your opposite hand could talk, it would be screaming, "put me in, coach!" For the most part, we have accepted the fact that we can only use one hand and one foot in this world. If you start working for your opposite hand, you will be amazed at the improvement! Throw a tennis ball against the wall, swing a baseball bat, tennis racquet, or golf club, or kick a soccer ball with your opposite limb. Before you know it, your lefty will start catching up to "old righty"; if you give it time, the lefty will start teaching the righty a few things. You've got to go lefty.

Capoeira

If you have never heard of Capoeira before, it is a martial art/dance form that has its origins in Africa and Brazil. Capoeira is another art you can plug into this system. Take a look at *The Little Capoeira Book*, by Nestor Capoeira. Consider it extra credit. If you decide to investigate this book, it will show you The *Ginga*, The *Negativa*, and The *Role* just to get you started. These three fabulous exercises are detailed for you in this great illustrated book by Nestor Capoeira, and you can **perform them on your mat.** Maybe you will walk further down the Capoeira roda? (Roda means *The Circle,* which is formed by Capoeirist musicians; inside the circle, two competing Capoerists meet to compete in the dance/martial art).

You may not have enough room on your mat to perform some of the advanced moves, but do what you can. Capoeira can help you develop strength, balance, and flexibility in another unique way.

There is a musical component to Capoeira: some song, and dance, a few musical instruments, a little poetry, and storytelling. Maybe that is why they are referred to as martial *artists*? I will not hesitate to place money on a martial artist with a background in Capoeira. I think there is a lot to be learned from this art.

I encourage you to take a step into the Capoeira structure. And start your workout with a little music and song. You don't have to play the berimbau, which is the lead instrument for Capoeira. Instead, sing your favorite song or dance your favorite dance or play your favorite instrument for just ten minutes before your exercise. It will loosen you up a tad and lift your spirits!

Run Swim Run

I would be remiss if I didn't share with you one of my favorite exercise routines. Make sure you have a good grasp of swimming before attempting this one. This routine, the famous run-swim-run one, is from *The Navy Seal Workout*, by Mark De Lisle. Begin with a ten-minute warm-up followed by a ten-minute run, a ten-minute swim, and finish with a ten-minute run. It's not quite the triangle training, but to quote Emerson, "a foolish consistency is the hobgoblin of little minds."

You can change it to a swim-run-swim or after speaking about it to a retired Navy Seal you may decide to try a run-swim-run-swim-run or a swim-run-swim-run-swim or even a swim-run-swim-run-swim-run. While doing your second run you might notice you're feeling a little better, or a little looser. The swim helps you stretch out a bit. It is always good to finish the day with some stretching, if you have the energy? The run-swim-run is a lotta fun!

Potluok

I think of a typical workout like a cook may think about preparing a meal or making a potluck. Imagine there are a few ingredients left in the kitchen, and we need to find the available ingredients to cook the day's potluck. I think of a workout in a similar way and like to grab different ingredients off the shelf in hopes of creating the perfect workout.

Or to think of it in a slightly different way, Jean Jacque Machado, a well-known martial artist, once wrote something to the effect of, you can draw up a certain move in martial arts, but that move is made in soft clay, meaning we can get creative and make changes that fit our particular bodies and abilities.

I have presented to you a basic format or a path to follow. You might even call it a yellow brick road because to follow this path, you will need some courage, some brains, and even a little heart (the heart is probably the most important, remember the Tin Man?) From here, I encourage you to add your favorite exercises and produce your favorite workout, and ideally have your spirit fly high in the sky!

The Way We Are Wired

Having a spinal injury has caused me to think about the way we are wired. It is apparent to me that the signals my brain sends to my limbs seem to be a little short-circuited. And that is why I struggle with things like balance. But it makes me wonder about other ways we are wired.

The first thing that comes to mind was the way my body cried out for food when I first began fasting. It would send out ferocious pangs, or seemingly demons, demanding that the body was fed. Now that I am a couple of years into a fasting routine, I enjoy going a day or so without food. I may feel a little discomfort from time to time, but I don't get the ferocious pangs anymore? It feels as if, in a way, I'm wired a little differently now.

Of course, another way we are wired is performing a simple skill like swimming. At first, I struggled to do the butterfly, but after continually attempting the stroke, my body and mind could eventually figure the stroke out. Now, years later, I'm wired for the butterfly.

Another example of being wired is playing the harmonica. If you decide to pick it up and learn a song, you will surprise yourself at some point. Start with a simple song like Happy Birthday. It's also a crowd pleaser! Once you learn it, you will never forget it. Playing the harmonica is almost as easy as humming the tune. It becomes imprinted on our brains. I could also refer to this process as downloading.

It's almost as if our consistent repetitions and our 30-minute practice sessions are downloading to our body and mind.

Another way I'm wired is anticipation. Before a workout, I know that I will feel good in just a short time. And I know that it will be an effortless process.

Thus, I tend to exercise more. I'm not wired to think that the workout today is going to be difficult. I anticipate a pleasurable relaxed experience.

And finally, through my experience, I came to understand how our spirit can be wired. Meaning if we decide to exercise, we will create a positive, optimistic spirit.

It's important to know that we are wired in these ways; so that we can be successful in any endeavor.

Let's take golf as an example. If you would like to be a successful golfer you need to hit golf balls 3 times a week for approximately 30 minutes each day. You might want to read a book or a pamphlet on the basics of the golf swing too, or watch YouTube videos?

Take baseball, tennis, soccer, the harmonica, the Hula Hoop, or any endeavor. Apply the same formula, and you will get proficient at that particular hobby. Once you really find out what you want to do, increase the frequency to every day for 30 minutes. To master a sport, you should practice twice a day. That's when you start thinking about taking off Sundays. And finally, when you become possessed and you want to be the best in the world, you move up to, all day, every day, sunup to sundown. I think that is how the yogis become so flexible?

While you are practicing your hobby, make sure to send the right message to your mind. Let's say you pull back an arrow and aim for the bull's eye. What message should go through your mind at this exact moment? Before you release the arrow, you should tell yourself, "I'm feeling good" or say, "I'm thankful for feeling good." At that moment, you can release the arrow and watch it fly to the target. If the arrow lands at the center of the bull's eye, you will feel good at that moment. If the arrow misses the target during one of your many practice shots, don't show frustration, anger, or disappointment. Instead, stay in the feel-good flow.

The Wall

If you have the time to get outside once in a while and would like to work on your coordination a little more, it would be great to find a wall that you can hit against. Maybe there is a wall at your local tennis court? It's not always easy to find a good wall. However, finding a good wall is like finding a good friend, and by spending time with this new friend, you will be rewarded.

Hitting against the wall can be as fun, as seen in the movie, "Field of Dreams." In the movie, a voice from the sky kept saying, "Build it, and he will come." If you keep hitting against the wall, listen to the voice that says, "hit against me and I will transform you." Baseball, cricket, tennis, soccer, lacrosse, hockey, handstands, and more... These are great ways of working on your opposite side, and your good side too!

Throwing the ball lefty and fielding the short hop barehanded is one of my all-time favorites.

Spend 30 minutes with the wall regularly, and you will be having too much fun! You might find yourself saying, "I feel like a million bucks."

Winning Feels Great!

One of the interesting things about the martial arts was the way winning made me feel. It's really difficult to describe the satisfaction of performing a submission in the martial arts. It takes a long time to figure it all out, and to perform your first submission feels good. Finally after a long period of time, the submissions start getting more frequent and you start applying many more submissions. To me it made sense that after a workout I would feel good. But the truth is if I had a good day on the mat, and put together some submissions I felt great! On the other hand, if I was submitted several times, despite the great workout, I did not feel that good.

Everyone loves to win, everyone loves a winner. We are actually wired to win, and I say this because no matter how lazy or tired I may have felt while grappling; when you feel that submission about to be applied you naturally give it "your all" to escape. I get that it's great to win, and it's important to win in this world. But what do you gain from losing? I think one of the great things about losing is your journey going back to the drawing board. Asking the questions: What did I do wrong? How can I get better? Maybe I should watch more videos, or read more books? Maybe I should exercise more, or exercise less, improve my diet, dive deeper? These are just a few of the questions you will ask yourself when you are a loser. And in a way, I think it is a good thing. I think this book is a compilation of the things I tried after losing, and the different ways I tried to improve myself. I truly believe there are some golden nuggets here if you are willing to sift through them.

Not everyone can win, at least half of us lose. Maybe after a win you will pop a bottle of champagne, but after a loss you will go back to the drawing board. I think there is something to be said for that.

Neuroscience and how it can help you

The disciplines in neuroscience are: mathematics, linguistics, engineering, computer science, chemistry, philosophy, psychology and medicine just to name a few.

Neuroscience is a fairly in depth subject matter; in its simplest form it includes: study of the nervous system which entails the study of your brain connected to neurons, axons, muscles or glands. Others may refer to this as a study of your body matrix, and it includes agility, balance and coordination; also proprioception the sense through which we perceive movement, position and allocated force. It also entails in its simplest form, learning the fundamentals of bioelectricity.

What does neuroscience tell us about learning different disciplines like music, mathematics, gymnastics, or languages?

If we know a little neuroscience it can help us achieve optimum learning. This is what neuroscience tells us about learning:

Learning involves changing the brain. Moderate stress is beneficial for learning. Mild and extreme stress are equally detrimental to learning. Adequate sleep, nutrition, and exercise encourage steady learning.

Active learning involves multiple neural connections in the brain for optimal learning to occur. For optimum learning the brain needs conditions which it is able to change in response to stimuli, and able to produce new neurons and create memory.

If the stress is too much we don't learn almost equally to the stress being too light. Moderate stress is optimal for learning.

This is one of the reasons why Feeling Good You recommends an intensity level of 50%. It produces optimum conditions for learning. We also feel that post workout your brain is at the ideal frequency for continued learning.

How do we learn from a scientific perspective to change the brain? We change the neural pathways. With consistent stimulation. Neural connections are strengthened by repetition creating neural pathways.

Consistent stimulation needs three regular controls: frequency, intensity and duration.

Feeling Good You prescribed method for change:

Frequency (everyday), intensity (moderate), duration (30 minutes).

After your workout the brain is at the optimum frequency to absorb information. If you follow this you can improve your ability to learn. Learning helps us feel good, improving at a skill helps us feel good, and to see steady improvement in any discipline can be very rewarding. Neuroscience can help us learn!

Make the Program Effortless

Many times, while watching a golfer, you can tell the moment a golf ball leaves the tee how capable the golfer is. If they look like they are trying to kill the ball and struggle to maintain good balance during their swing. They might have their troubles on the course.

However, if they have a swing that looks effortless, they are probably a superior golfer with a low handicap. A basketball shot is similar in that you can tell that the beautiful relaxed **effortless** shot is more than likely going in. Let's look at competitive swimming as an example. When Mark Spitz won his Olympic gold medals, he seemingly had an effortless stroke.

To help find the effortless state of mind, start with walking. While taking a leisurely 30-minute walk look for the perfect rhythm, the perfect breath (nasal breathing with Darth Vader breathing), the perfect length of your step, the right pulse or heart rate, and the perfect balance in every step.

When you find this relaxed effortless state, and you feel as if you are gliding along the path, you are in the flow.

Try to incorporate this state in all your exercises. Performing qigong and ballet will help you manifest an effortless state. Add a little beauty, and a little flow, into all your workouts.

Look, listen and feel

The feel-good spirit can be a little allusive at times. Maybe you finish your workout and feel better than you did the day before, and some days you don't. Some days you will feel better than other days and that is to be expected. Personally, when it comes to feeling good, I get my best results with swimming. Seemingly, I feel great every time I leave the pool! Handstands also tend to help me feel particularly good. Someone else may prefer yoga, Pilates, or running. We are all different. If you do not hit your target heart rate during a workout and feel the need to do so, choose your favorite strength or cardio exercises like, the push-up, the Hula Hoop, or kettlebell, and hit the target rate just once during the 30 minutes. The point is to look, listen and feel to figure out what triggers the fix for you, how long you should stay near the target, or how many times you can hit the target heart rate to feel your best.

Pay attention to how you feel throughout the day. You may feel extra good after an extremely vigorous workout. The downside could be that you crash shortly after the workout and spend the rest of your day napping. On the other hand, if you are young with high energy and willing to take some risks, you may decide to try a martial art or something where you can push yourself to higher heights and take it to the limit!

Breathing and Lung Capacity

One last thing about breathing. Maybe we have gone a little overboard on this breathing stuff? However, when it comes to athletics, breathing or your lung capacity is often the key. You may see in the first round of a boxing match, one particular fighter seems to outclass the other fighter. However, towards the end of the second round, things might start going the other way because the other fighter has more endurance and better cardio. And the longer the fight goes on the more apparent it becomes that the less skilled fighter has more staying power or spirit. What he lacks in skill he makes up in breathing ability.

Breath is also important for world-class marksmen. Being a great sniper or shooting a bow and arrow has a lot to do with a rehearsed breathing technique and being still.

Some people say that life starts with the baby's first breath at birth, and it ends with the last gasp of breath, away goes the spirit. The breath and the spirit are interconnected and as we exercise to strengthen our breath, we strengthen our spirit. My sensei once told us that to be successful at martial arts, you have to dive deep. I really wasn't sure what he meant, but at that moment it was almost as if he were saying, "dive deep grasshopper." I started to think about it and when I looked around at the class it became pretty obvious to me that the people who were successful at martial arts really put their time in. They went to the morning classes; they went to the evening classes; they studied tapes and memorized the seemingly endless moves. What I'm trying to say is that when it comes to this breathing stuff you may have to do your homework to get it right, and it may take some time. As your breathing improves you will realize it is sort of a sinus thing where you finally open up your sinuses and you can breathe through your nose. Low and behold, you will discover that this is your most important asset as an athlete.

It is also important for those of us working on just staying alive!

The good thing is we are going to feel good and look good before we master our breathing. It would be nice if we could develop our breathing capacity to the point where we can run a marathon or a triathlon while breathing through our nose the whole time. I'm not expecting you to reach that point, but it is nice to have goals and to reach for the sky. What I would like you to be able to do is carry your groceries into the house while breathing through your nose. Studies show that most people are mouth breathers; and because we have become mouth breathers we have lost the ability to breathe easily through our noses.

Here are a couple of keys to unlocking your nose in the beginning:

1. Purchase the Breathe-Right strips. They are like band-aids that cover your nose and open your nostrils.

2. Start doing a nasal rinse. I recommend Neal Med; it is an all-natural product.

3. Perform The Sun Salutation, it will help open your sinuses.

4. Foods that open up your sinuses, like kimchi, horseradish, or red-hot chili peppers, are good. Hot showers, steam baths, and Vick's will also help.

5. Drink "Breathe Deep" herbal tea, by Yogi. Every tea bag comes with yogi words of wisdom, here is one: "Your breath fills you with energy, anywhere and anytime you need it."

When you are performing yoga, it is good to find your stretching number. Take note of how many breaths or seconds it takes until you start unlocking your muscles and you can stretch that extra inch or so? It's good to know that number and to experiment at times with different numbers to see if another number might work better for you or unlock your muscles even further. I know we have a limited amount of time to exercise, but assuming we have the extra time this is a fun and interesting game to play. When we reach those higher numbers, we not only unlock our muscles, but we can unlock our sinuses too.

Another number that you should search for is your recovery number. How many Darth Vader breaths does it take for you to start feeling relaxed and recovered during the peak of your workout? These numbers will change over time as you get more conditioned; when in doubt, take a few extra breaths.

And finally, don't underestimate the power of the harmonica. Simply put, playing the harmonica helps improve lung function, and it works muscles in and around your lungs that regular exercise cannot.

No Pain No Gain

Remember the old slogan, "no pain no gain." That was the mantra years ago when the gym teachers would have us give a hundred and ten percent when doing our workouts. Run as fast as you can, lift as much weight as you can, do all repetitions to failure. No pain no gain…give it all you have. Go, go, go, go, go! Whistle!

I think it is important to note that the first time, after my accident, that I remember feeling or recognizing the spirit, the positive, feel-good, SGPR High, Soaring Spirit I was surfing a longboard dragging my hand along the wall of a wave. Although surfing may look pretty laid back it takes a significant amount of effort to paddle out to the wave, and then paddle to catch the wave, let alone stand up, keep your balance, and ride the wave out. Chances are you are giving *your all* to catch that wave.

In the martial arts gym, I recognized the spirit frequently after my first spar. While practicing self-defense odds are you are exercising close to your maximum capacity. After martial arts, I began to search for the feel-good spirit in yoga, Pilates, ballet, and the Genius of Flexibility. Eventually, I was able to increase the good vibrations by adding strength and cardio exercises. The real revelation was when I discovered the art of controlling my heart rate by keeping the pulse at or below the 50% exertion rate. Where previously to feel good my heart rate was typically at its maximum rate. Now, I barely break a sweat and I have the luxury of being able to find or manufacture the exercise high or "the fix" with minimal effort. Which makes this the great lazy person's workout! It's really just about effortless. No pain and strain, just gain, or "relax and enjoy your workout" is the new mantra.

The Supercalifragilistic 9-minute workout!

I started by telling you I had a thirty-minute workout that will make you look good and feel good too, but I like to under-promise and over-deliver.

What we can do as well is The Great, Supercalifragilistic 9-minute workout. To do the great nine-minute workout start with the Sun Salute for 5 minutes or swing an Indian Club? After this warm-up, choose your favorite vigorous exercise and hit your target heart rate in 1- 3 minutes. To finish, jump in the shower for one minute, try the Scottish shower for 30 seconds like James Bond. That's all you need to do, to look good and feel good too!

Where are we, and where are we going when it comes to fitness?

I don't know where you are when it comes to fitness. Maybe you are someone who has never exercised before or dieted. Maybe you are a world champion at some type of sport. The point is whatever your level of fitness, it's our objective to find ourselves. Maybe we should just do the Supercalifragilistic 9-minute workout three times a week. That's the easiest path and we will look good and feel good too!

Maybe we want a little more.

Perhaps, we want to lower our golf handicap or get better at tennis? Maybe we'd like to fit into our wedding dress. Whatever our goals are determines how much time we will spend on the path, and which direction we will take. Find a comfortable, relaxed pace, and don't forget to smell the roses.

Meditation – Exercise for your mind.

In my opinion, the best time to meditate is immediately after you exercise and shower. By exercising your body first, you will bathe your mind with positive emotions and be able to focus or meditate in a good frame of mind. Listening to music that induces brain waves like binaural beats, or simply sounds of nature can be helpful. Actually practicing a musical instrument can be considered a form of meditation, and it can help change your state of mind. A great place to meditate is on your mat, you can start by sitting American Indian style, or sitting in the Lotus position. To investigate meditation, look in the *Qigong Bible* by Katherine Allen, and read the chapter entitled Qigong Meditation. The Yoga books will also help, and B.K.S Iyengar can give expert advice about meditation.

I also suggest you pick up a copy of *Think and Grow Rich* by Napoleon Hill. If you follow the suggestions in this book you will need to visualize and control your mind by filling it only with positive affirmations. You can take this book, and its philosophy seriously by studying it every day for 30 minutes. In order to manifest money you will need to meditate on this book's instructions. Making money feels good. To find more information and to learn more about how to think and grow rich watch the movie: Think and Grow Rich The Movie at *Thinkandgrowrichyou.com.*

To contact a mentor that can show you the secrets of making money, and get you feeling good; you can contact *Livingthelegacyyou.com*.

The Power of Positive Thinking by Norman Vincent Peale is another favorite self-help book that encourages you to empty your mind and think positively. He also suggests that a great way to meditate is to sit in a rocking chair and feel the warmth of the sun.

A final note on fasting.

I have spent the majority of this eBook talking about exercise, but I'd like to remind you that for years I exercised at a vigorous pace for 2 hours at a time, three times a week and I looked *Shlobby*. After doing the moderate exercises demonstrated in this work for 30 minutes, every other day, and fasting twice a week for a few months, my new nickname was Slim-Jim. My point is no matter how hard you exercise, if you eat too much you are going to be overweight, and not up to snuff. One of the secrets to maintaining this diet is the Bragg apple cider vinegar cocktail, which is 8 oz. of water, a tablespoon of apple cider vinegar, and a tablespoon of honey. Drinking this cocktail when you are hungry instead of having a meal is a great way to reduce your calories. I find the ACV cocktail to be very satisfying and it helps you go a few hours before your next meal. Having just a morsel of honey seems to always satisfy my sweet tooth. And it seems like the honey along with the apple cider vinegar provides an abundance of energy.

The reason this program works and I can promise that you will look good and feel good too with only 9-minute and 30-minute workouts, is in great part because of the fasting routine. I try to go without the ACV cocktail when I fast, but if I feel too uncomfortable and notice a headache or a severe lack of energy, on occasions, I will drink the cocktail while fasting to help make it through. This is a nice crutch to use when you first begin fasting. During many of my fasts, I feel great and look forward to the fasting days as my favorite days, and without a doubt, I have the most enjoyable suppers!

Finding the Path.

When you realize you can feel your best through exercise and wash away the negative emotions, and when you can achieve the exercise high in 30 minutes or less, you are on the right path.

We are manufacturing a good spirit, and you will feel the joy when you start doing these simple 30-minute workouts at home.

Don't forget to clean your mat! When you find happiness in cleaning your mat, you're on your way.

Granted, I threw a few books at you and you did have to do some homework. We even did some painstaking math, but after completing this work, even scoring a D- with minimal effort, I believe you will say it was worth it. You won't fail, and you will transform.

And you will begin to appreciate the little things a little more.

1,2,3, Go!

Can we now pan to a stretch limousine driving off into the sunset or should we just YouTube the final scene of Trading Places starring Eddie Murphy and Dan Aykroyd? I think you get the idea.

Looking good, Billy Ray....

Feeling good, Louis!

You are on your own now...Adios Amigo or Amiga! My friend! Stay on the Supercalifragilistic, Great, Pure, Righteous, High, Soaring Spirits path!

Go now, and start **FeelingGoodYou!**

Thank you for reviewing this book!

Reviews make the publishing world go round. You can review this book on Amazon…Thank you!!!

Suggested Resources

I am not endorsing the advice in any of these books, but I did find these books personally helpful.

Suggested Books

1. *Eat Stop Eat* by Brad Pilon

2. *The Miracle of Fasting* by Patricia Bragg N.D., Ph.D. & Paul Bragg N. D., Ph.D.

3. *Body, Mind, and Sport* by John Douillard

4. *Genius of Flexibility* by Bob Cooley

5. *The Illustrated Light on Yoga* by B. K. S. Iyengar

6. *Yoga the Iyengar Way, The New Definitive Illustrated Guide* by Silva, Mira & Shyam Mehta

7. *The Pilates Powerhouse* by Mari Winsor

8. *The New York City Ballet Workout* by Peter Martins

9. *Qigong Bible* by Katherine Allen

Extra Books

10. *The Navy Seal Workout: The Complete Total Body Fitness Program* by Mark De Lisle

11. *The Little Capoeira Book* by Nelson Capoeira

12. *Total Immersion* by Terry Laughlin

13. *The Power of Positive Thinking* by Norman Vincent Peale

14. *Think and Grow Rich* by Napoleon Hill

15. *What Would Jesus Eat* by Don Colbert, M.D

16. *The Vegetarian Female* by Anika Avery Grant, RD

17. *Superfoods* by Robin Keuneke

18. *Extra Lean* by Mario Lopez

19. *The Collagen Diet* by Pamela Schoenfeld, MS, RD, LDN

20. *The Best of Chief Dan George* by Chief Dan George

21. *How to Play Harmonica* by Marcos Habif

22. *The Art of The Short Game* by Stan Utley

23. *Harvey Penick's Little Red Book: Lessons And Teachings From A Lifetime in Golf* by Harvey Penick

24. *The Magic* by Rhonda Byrne

25. *Knee Ability Zero* by Ben Patrick

Suggested Purchases

To get started:

- 2 yoga mats, maybe 3?
- 1 6'x9' exercise mat or just a king-size blanket, a comforter, or a rug to get started.
- 1 10-pound kettlebell
- 1 pull-up bar
- 1 16 oz. water bottle
- 1 pair of swim goggles
- 1 box of earplugs (**be very careful with earplugs; always read the directions**)
- 1 swim cap
- 1 bathing suit
- 1 towel
- 1 long underwear top and bottom (I use and recommend Bodtek)

Extra Purchases

- Hula Hoop
- Sidewinder
- Stretch n flex
- 1 pair of Indian Clubs, 2 pounds
- Vitamin C
- Apple cider vinegar
- NutriBullet
- Vinegar (for cleaning the mats)
- Water delivery service

Made in the USA
Columbia, SC
16 September 2022

67415192R00041